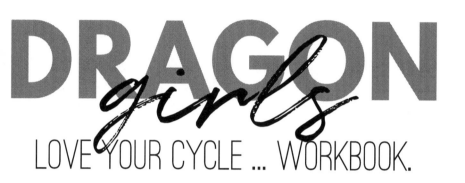

CELESTE CAMPBELL

THIS WORKBOOK IS A COMPANION TO
DRAGON GIRLS
LOVE YOUR CYCLE ... PERIOD.

HOW TO USE THIS BOOK

The key to accessing the power of your dragons is getting to know them individually. You can do this by tracking your cycle and then looking for patterns on each day of your cycle. This workbook is designed to help you accomplish that goal.

The steps are simple:

1. On the first day of your cycle, or the first day you bleed, open up to the page labeled "Day 1." If you don't menstruate or have an irregular cycle, start on the first day of the new moon.

2. Write down a few observations about the day in the square labeled "Cycle 1."

Cycle 1 You can write the date here.   **DAY 1.**

This is where you will write a few observations about the day. This is not a journal - you do not have to make a full account of everything that happened or your profound thoughts during the day. Take just a few minutes to write down observations about your mood, behavior, your level of menstrual pain, or anything else of interest.

3. On the next day, open to the next page labeled "Day 2."

4. Repeat step 2, but write observations for Day 2.

5. Repeat this process until you bleed again. This workbook provides pages until day 35. If you haven't bled again, that means your cycle is irregular. Don't worry too much about that, especially if you have only recently begun your cycle. If you do have any concerns about that, consult a trusted adult or a doctor.

6. When you bleed again, or on the next new moon, return to the page labeled "Day 1."

DAY 1.

Cycle 2

At this point, don't make any judgments about your cycle. You are still in the observation phase. Write about your experience on this day, just like you did last time.

7. Repeat until you have made observations about your cycle until you have filled out the section labeled "Cycle 5" on the last day of your cycle. This should take you about five months to do.

8. On Day 1 of your sixth cycle, open up to Day 1 once more. Answer the questions on the right side of the page. These questions will prompt you to look for patterns in yourself. Feel free to deviate from the questions, or even answer them in another notebook so that you have more room to think about it.

What patterns do you see on this day of your cycle?

Remember this activity is about gathering information that could better your life. Avoiding using negative language to describe your body or behavior.

9. Continue this process until you have analyzed all the days of your cycle.

10. Congratulations! You now have a user manual that will help you make decisions about how to plan your life.

11. Don't stop tracking your cycle. Either get another copy of this tracker, or keep tracking in another notebook. You will always have more to learn about your body and more ways you can improve!

DAY 1 EXAMPLE.

Cycle 1

I felt connected today. I had so many thoughts and inspirations running around inside my mind. I decided to journal about it and wow, it was a great session. My pain was pretty mild today. I took a bath and drank some tea and took it really easy. I was also tired all day.

Cycle 2

I was happy and in a great mood today... just achy and lethargic. I didn't want to do much except lay around today. I wanted to journal but it was hard to convince myself to do it.

Cycle 3

Strangely enough, I felt kind of hyper today. I went and visited some friends and I felt really happy to be around them. I did start to feel pretty tired when I got home though so I took it easy the rest of the day. The pain started after I got home and was uncomfortable but mild.

Cycle 4

Today I had a full day of activities planned, and I did okay, but was so exhausted by the end of it. I started even feeling a little moody by the end of the day. I normally feel recharged when I spend time around people, but today it was hard.

Cycle 5

I felt super meh today. My pain was REALLY bad in the middle of the night. I had a hard time sleeping. I have been a little more stressed than normal so that's probably why. It's also been really busy the last few days. I have been having a lot of existential thoughts all day today.

What patterns do you see on this day of your cycle?

I have noticed that, while I might expect day one of my cycle to be a struggle, I'm usually really happy. Lethargic, but happy. It's hard to motivate myself to do anything. I get tired really quickly. I also notice that my pain is significantly lessened when I take it easy the days before I start bleeding.

What activities feel the best for you on this day?

I have noticed that when I can motivate myself to journal, I am very thoughtful and creative. It can be hard to motivate myself to do so, but it's so worth it. My pain is lessened when I do things to restore myself, such as taking a bath, drinking tea, or reading.

How can you better care for yourself on this day? Do you have any other observations?

It's very tempting to sit and scroll on my phone all day. But that doesn't actually make me feel any better. I think if I put my phone in the cupboard, it will help me to actually rest and restore because it won't be available. I love taking baths and drinking tea on this day, but it's really hard to motivate myself to put those together. So I think if I have them prepped and ready to go before I start bleeding, that will really help. I'll also be sure and get my journal all picked out, find a working pen, and pick out a reading book a few days before day one.

AFFIRMATIONS

Before each set of seven days, this book includes affirmations for the season. If your seasons vary in length by a few days, don't worry. You are whole exactly as you are!

Your sub conscience is very powerful. Its job is to do exactly what you tell it to do. As you speak kindly to yourself, your thoughts about yourself will change over time.

You can use these affirmations during each season to remind yourself of your journey. If you find yourself having negative feelings toward your body at any point, try looking at yourself in the mirror and saying these affirmations to yourself 3 times.

You may also come up with your own statements. Use present statements like "I am," "I have," "I do," instead of "I will," or "I want to." Use statements that make you feel empowered.

If you find it difficult to say an affirmation, it might be because you don't believe what you are saying. If this happens, you can try replacing the statement "I am…" with "I am open to becoming…" For example, instead of saying "I am beautiful." Say "I am open to seeing my own beauty." Over time, you will become more conformable with the idea of saying "I am beautiful." Work toward using the "I am" statement.

MAKE YOURSELF *a priority*

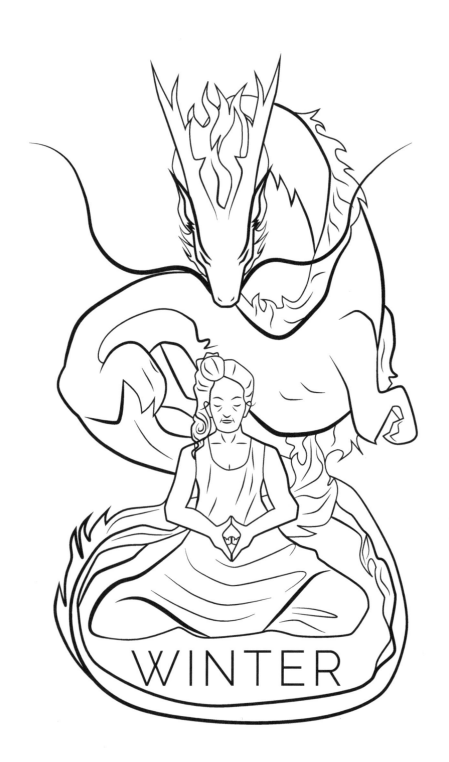

WINTER
The Bleed

I AM MY OWN BEST CARETAKER

I KNOW WHAT MY BODY NEEDS

I AM GRATEFUL FOR MY BODY AND ALL IT DOES FOR ME

I AM A CREATOR

THE CYCLE OF CREATION EXISTS WITHIN ME

Here's an extra space for notes

Notes

DAY 1.

Cycle 1

Cycle 2

Cycle 3

Cycle 4

Cycle 5

What patterns do you see on this day of your cycle?

What activities feel the best for you on this day?

How can you better care for yourself on this day?
Do you have any other observations?

DAY 2.

Cycle 1

Cycle 2

Cycle 3

Cycle 4

Cycle 5

What patterns do you see on this day of your cycle?

What activities feel the best for you on this day?

How can you better care for yourself on this day?
Do you have any other observations?

DAY 3.

Cycle 1

Cycle 2

Cycle 3

Cycle 4

Cycle 5

What patterns do you see on this day of your cycle?

What activities feel the best for you on this day?

How can you better care for yourself on this day?
Do you have any other observations?

DAY 4.

Cycle 1

Cycle 2

Cycle 3

Cycle 4

Cycle 5

What patterns do you see on this day of your cycle?

What activities feel the best for you on this day?

How can you better care for yourself on this day?
Do you have any other observations?

DAY 5.

Cycle 1

Cycle 2

Cycle 3

Cycle 4

Cycle 5

What patterns do you see on this day of your cycle?

What activities feel the best for you on this day?

How can you better care for yourself on this day?
Do you have any other observations?

DAY 6.

Cycle 1

Cycle 2

Cycle 3

Cycle 4

Cycle 5

What patterns do you see on this day of your cycle?

What activities feel the best for you on this day?

How can you better care for yourself on this day?
Do you have any other observations?

DAY 7.

Cycle 1

Cycle 2

Cycle 3

Cycle 4

Cycle 5

What patterns do you see on this day of your cycle?

What activities feel the best for you on this day?

How can you better care for yourself on this day?
Do you have any other observations?

LOVE YOURSELF
AS YOU ARE
right now

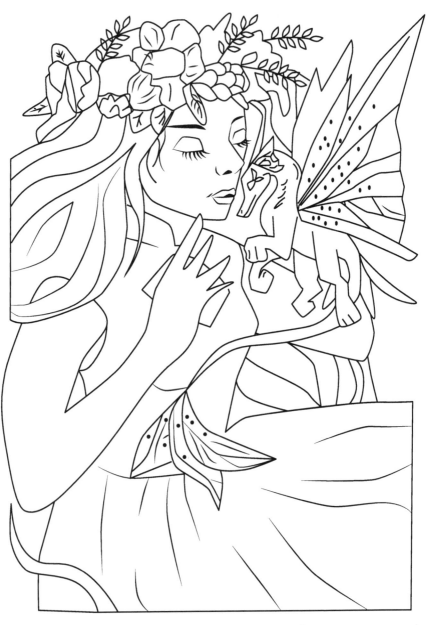

SPRING

SPRING *rebirth*

I ACCOMPLISH MY GOALS

I CREATE SUCCESS IN MY LIFE

I AM GRATEFUL FOR EVERY MOMENT

I SPEAK MY TRUTH

I EMBRACE DISCOMFORT
IN ORDER TO CREATE POSITIVE CHANGE IN LIFE

I LOVE EVERYONE AND EVERYONE LOVES ME

DAY 8.

Cycle 1

Cycle 2

Cycle 3

Cycle 4

Cycle 5

What patterns do you see on this day of your cycle?

What activities feel the best for you on this day?

How can you better care for yourself on this day?
Do you have any other observations?

DAY 9.

Cycle 1

Cycle 2

Cycle 3

Cycle 4

Cycle 5

What patterns do you see on this day of your cycle?

What activities feel the best for you on this day?

How can you better care for yourself on this day?
Do you have any other observations?

DAY 10.

Cycle 1

Cycle 2

Cycle 3

Cycle 4

Cycle 5

What patterns do you see on this day of your cycle?

What activities feel the best for you on this day?

How can you better care for yourself on this day?
Do you have any other observations?

DAY 11.

Cycle 1

Cycle 2

Cycle 3

Cycle 4

Cycle 5

What patterns do you see on this day of your cycle?

What activities feel the best for you on this day?

How can you better care for yourself on this day?
Do you have any other observations?

DAY 12.

Cycle 1

Cycle 2

Cycle 3

Cycle 4

Cycle 5

What patterns do you see on this day of your cycle?

What activities feel the best for you on this day?

How can you better care for yourself on this day?
Do you have any other observations?

DAY 13.

Cycle 1

Cycle 2

Cycle 3

Cycle 4

Cycle 5

What patterns do you see on this day of your cycle?

What activities feel the best for you on this day?

How can you better care for yourself on this day?
Do you have any other observations?

DAY 14.

Cycle 1

Cycle 2

Cycle 3

Cycle 4

Cycle 5

What patterns do you see on this day of your cycle?

What activities feel the best for you on this day?

How can you better care for yourself on this day?
Do you have any other observations?

REMINDER...

These next few pages represent the summer of the cycle. Here's a friendly reminder not to "should" all over yourself. Your task is to make observations about your mood and behavior in order to look for patterns. Maybe you don't feel that "big summer energy" during this phase. That's okay! By making observations, you may find that you actually get burst of energy during a different phase of your cycle.

It is possible that you won't experience certain energies during your cycle because of outside factors. Stress, for example, will most definitely impact your cycle.

There are a hundred thousand self help books out there about how to live a better life. It's easy to get swept up in the overload of information. By paying attention to your cycle, you will be able to personalize your self care. You will never know what exactly is helping you and hurting you until you pay attention.

Take a deep breath. Observation is the first step.

You are
ENOUGH

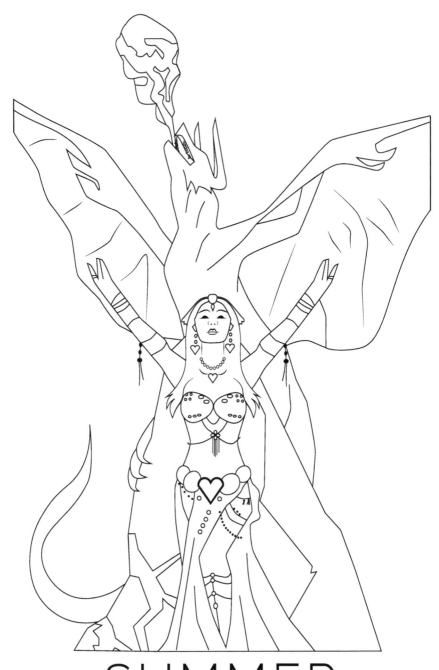

SUMMER *ovulation*

I AM WILD AND FREE

I EMBRACE MY INNER FLAME

I AM A CHILD AT HEART

I AM DIVINELY BEAUTIFUL

I AM JOY

I LOVE MY BODY

DAY 15.

Cycle 1

Cycle 2

Cycle 3

Cycle 4

Cycle 5

What patterns do you see on this day of your cycle?

What activities feel the best for you on this day?

How can you better care for yourself on this day?
Do you have any other observations?

DAY 16.

Cycle 1

Cycle 2

Cycle 3

Cycle 4

Cycle 5

What patterns do you see on this day of your cycle?

What activities feel the best for you on this day?

How can you better care for yourself on this day?
Do you have any other observations?

DAY 17.

Cycle 1

Cycle 2

Cycle 3

Cycle 4

Cycle 5

What patterns do you see on this day of your cycle?

What activities feel the best for you on this day?

How can you better care for yourself on this day?
Do you have any other observations?

DAY 18.

Cycle 1

Cycle 2

Cycle 3

Cycle 4

Cycle 5

What patterns do you see on this day of your cycle?

What activities feel the best for you on this day?

How can you better care for yourself on this day?
Do you have any other observations?

DAY 19.

Cycle 1

Cycle 2

Cycle 3

Cycle 4

Cycle 5

What patterns do you see on this day of your cycle?

What activities feel the best for you on this day?

How can you better care for yourself on this day?
Do you have any other observations?

DAY 20.

Cycle 1

Cycle 2

Cycle 3

Cycle 4

Cycle 5

What patterns do you see on this day of your cycle?

What activities feel the best for you on this day?

How can you better care for yourself on this day?
Do you have any other observations?

DAY 21.

Cycle 1

Cycle 2

Cycle 3

Cycle 4

Cycle 5

What patterns do you see on this day of your cycle?

What activities feel the best for you on this day?

How can you better care for yourself on this day?
Do you have any other observations?

LOVE
who you are

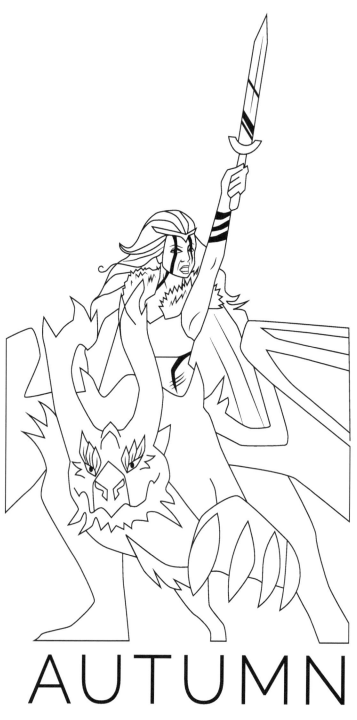

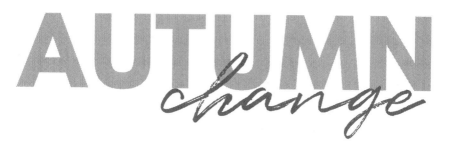

AUTUMN *change*

MY FEELINGS ARE VALID

I MANAGE MY EMOTIONS IN HEALTHY WAYS

I LOVE WHO I AM BECOMING

I EMBRACE THE FULL SPECTRUM OF MY FEELINGS

I CHANGE THE WORLD FOR THE BETTER

Notes

Notes

Cycle 1

Cycle 2

Cycle 3

Cycle 4

Cycle 5

DAY 22.

What patterns do you see on this day of your cycle?

What activities feel the best for you on this day?

How can you better care for yourself on this day?
Do you have any other observations?

DAY 23.

Cycle 1

Cycle 2

Cycle 3

Cycle 4

Cycle 5

What patterns do you see on this day of your cycle?

What activities feel the best for you on this day?

How can you better care for yourself on this day?
Do you have any other observations?

DAY 24.

Cycle 1

Cycle 2

Cycle 3

Cycle 4

Cycle 5

What patterns do you see on this day of your cycle?

What activities feel the best for you on this day?

How can you better care for yourself on this day?
Do you have any other observations?

DAY 25.

Cycle 1

Cycle 2

Cycle 3

Cycle 4

Cycle 5

What patterns do you see on this day of your cycle?

What activities feel the best for you on this day?

How can you better care for yourself on this day?
Do you have any other observations?

DAY 26.

Cycle 1

Cycle 2

Cycle 3

Cycle 4

Cycle 5

What patterns do you see on this day of your cycle?

What activities feel the best for you on this day?

How can you better care for yourself on this day?
Do you have any other observations?

DAY 27.

Cycle 1

Cycle 2

Cycle 3

Cycle 4

Cycle 5

What patterns do you see on this day of your cycle?

What activities feel the best for you on this day?

How can you better care for yourself on this day?
Do you have any other observations?

DAY 28.

Cycle 1

Cycle 2

Cycle 3

Cycle 4

Cycle 5

What patterns do you see on this day of your cycle?

What activities feel the best for you on this day?

How can you better care for yourself on this day?
Do you have any other observations?

You are the
REAL THING

Notes

Notes

DAY 29.

Cycle 1

Cycle 2

Cycle 3

Cycle 4

Cycle 5

What patterns do you see on this day of your cycle?

What activities feel the best for you on this day?

How can you better care for yourself on this day?
Do you have any other observations?

DAY 30.

Cycle 1

Cycle 2

Cycle 3

Cycle 4

Cycle 5

What patterns do you see on this day of your cycle?

What activities feel the best for you on this day?

How can you better care for yourself on this day?
Do you have any other observations?

DAY 31.

Cycle 1

Cycle 2

Cycle 3

Cycle 4

Cycle 5

What patterns do you see on this day of your cycle?

What activities feel the best for you on this day?

How can you better care for yourself on this day?
Do you have any other observations?

DAY 32.

Cycle 1

Cycle 2

Cycle 3

Cycle 4

Cycle 5

What patterns do you see on this day of your cycle?

What activities feel the best for you on this day?

How can you better care for yourself on this day?
Do you have any other observations?

DAY 33.

Cycle 1

Cycle 2

Cycle 3

Cycle 4

Cycle 5

What patterns do you see on this day of your cycle?

What activities feel the best for you on this day?

How can you better care for yourself on this day?
Do you have any other observations?

DAY 34.

Cycle 1

Cycle 2

Cycle 3

Cycle 4

Cycle 5

What patterns do you see on this day of your cycle?

What activities feel the best for you on this day?

How can you better care for yourself on this day?
Do you have any other observations?

DAY 35.

Cycle 1

Cycle 2

Cycle 3

Cycle 4

Cycle 5

What patterns do you see on this day of your cycle?

What activities feel the best for you on this day?

How can you better care for yourself on this day?
Do you have any other observations?

Notes

Notes

Notes

Notes

Notes

Notes

A SHAMELESS PLUG

I am extremely passionate about helping people discover their potential. I feel that the message in my book is one that can help heal the world in many ways. It's really not just for women. We all have work to do in learning to love ourselves. I have created a few additional resources that can act as companions to this book.

- A Facebook group just for girls and women to be safe to openly talk about their experience with their cycles! It's free to join! Just search for Dragon Girls on Facebook! (There's also a group for mamas! Search Dragon Mamas!)

- Affirmation cards - these are prints of the four dragons with affirmations listed on the back for each stage of the cycle.

You can find these resources and links on my website. By signing up for my email newsletter, you will stay up to date on all my projects. (For there will be many!) **thedragongrl.com**

I give presentations and offer a course on this topic! Feel free to contact me for more information!

Made in the USA
Middletown, DE
02 May 2022